MARIA CIANCIOLO

DEMENTIA CAREGIVING 101

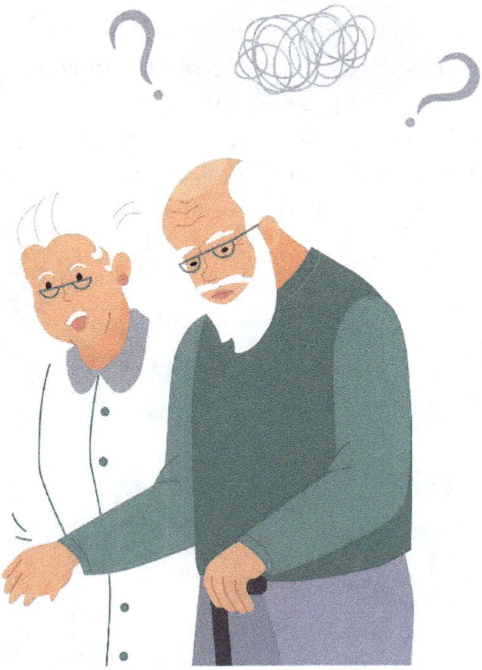

Dedicated To

Donna L. Cianciolo

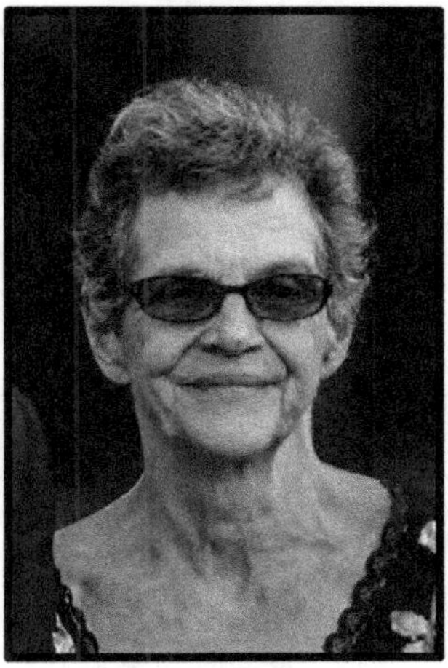

whose life and courage with Alzheimer's
continue to guide and inspire
those she left behind.
Her resilience in the face of Alzheimer's
taught me that
Love and Inspiration never fade...

CONTENTS

INTRODUCTION

WHY WRITE A RESOURCE GUIDE FOR FAMILY MEMBERS & CAREGIVERS?

I chose to write a resource guide for family members and caregivers about dementia called "Kaleidoscope" because a term "kaleidoscope" is a metaphor often used in the context of aging and caregiving. It describes the ever-changing pattern of experiences, needs, and emotions involved in the journey.

This guide would provide a roadmap for family members and caregivers, helping them navigate the diverse and evolving challenges of dementia care, offering support, information, and a sense of community.

Key reasons and themes for using the "Kaleidoscope" metaphor in such a guide include:

- **Reflecting the changing journey:** The term highlights that the experience of dementia care is not a straight path through predictable stages, but a series of twists and turns, with conditions and needs constantly shifting.

- **Highlighting diverse experiences:** Just as a kaleidoscope contains a diverse collection of elements, the guide acknowledges the varied perspectives of individuals with dementia, their family members, friends, and healthcare professionals.

- **Providing perspective and reframing:** The guide encourages caregivers to "turn the kaleidoscope lens" to see life in a new way, adapt to new realities, find moments of joy, and manage the "swirling emotions" that accompany the disease.

- **Offering a "treasure" of information:** The guide is intended to be a comprehensive and practical resource, a "mixed bag" or "treasure" of information to help reduce stress, enhance quality of life, and connect families with valuable community and professional resources.

- **Empowerment and advocacy:** The guide aims to empower family members and caregivers with practical knowledge and tools to advocate for appropriate healthcare and support services, ensuring the individual with dementia can live with dignity.

Ultimately, the guide uses the metaphor of a kaleidoscope to frame the complex and often overwhelming experience of dementia care as something that, while challenging, can reveal new perspectives and provide moments of beauty and connection when viewed through an informed and supportive lens.

WHY TITLE THE GUIDE "KALEIDOSCOPE"?

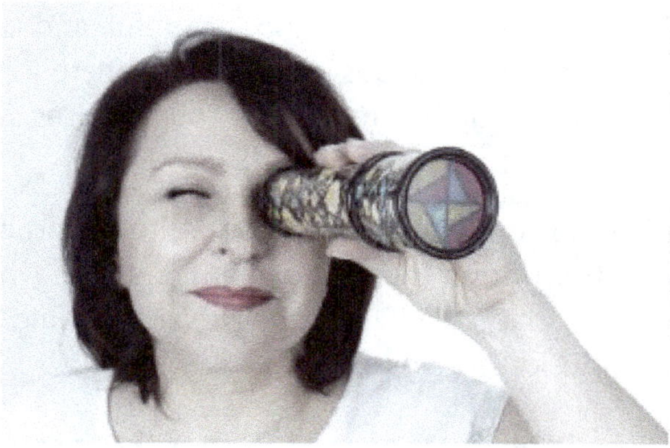

Figure 1 Kaleidoscope

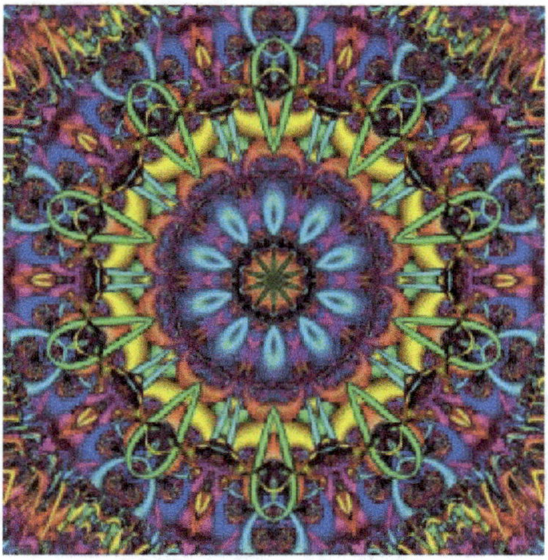

Figure 2 Kaleidoscopic View

The word "**Kaleidoscope**" literally means "observer of beautiful things" or "an instrument for seeing beautiful shapes," from the Greek words kalos (beautiful), eidos (shape), and-scope (an instrument for seeing).

What does this have to do with dementia?

Well, it symbolizes ever-changing, beautiful, and complex patterns formed by changes in the brain. Where they were once able to control their responses and impulses, they are no longer able to.

I visualize the colored glass, as their attitude and choices. The light transforms them into unique, shifting designs, highlighting adaptability, perspective, and finding beauty amidst confusion and loss.

The 4 Key interpretation of Dementia through the kaleidoscope:

Validation: Dementia presents patterns constantly; living moment to moment, what was true yesterday will change today requiring us to adapt and live in their moment (validate).

Control Your View: We can't choose the "glass" (changes in the brain) but we control the "light" (our positivity and approaches) to see beauty in the patterns.

Embrace Change: Our eyes are the instrument to observe the person with dementia when the illness is progressing.

Basic Human Needs: love, safety, warmth, hunger, security, reassurance, hope and purpose

CHAPTER 1

WHAT IS DEMENTIA?

It's an umbrella term used to describe a range of neurological conditions affecting the brain that worsens over time.

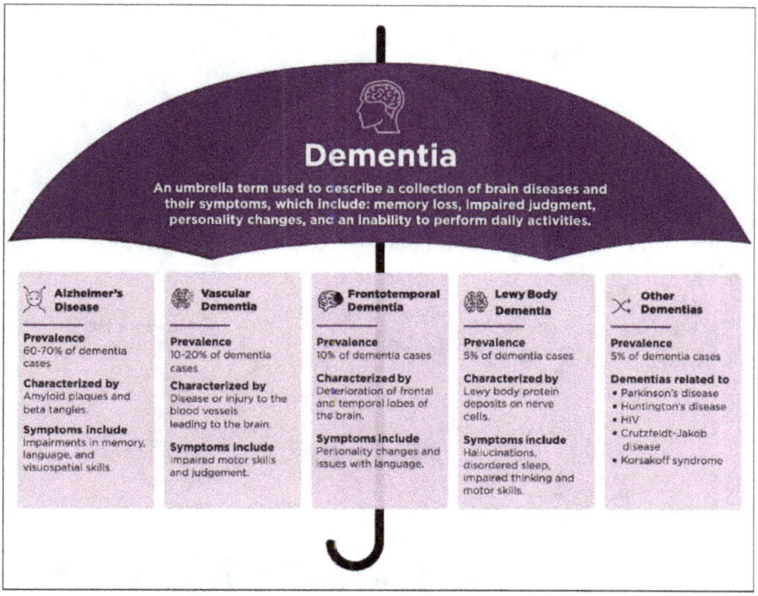

It is the loss of ability to think, remember, and reason to levels that affect daily life and activities. In the past, dementia was sometimes referred to as "senility' and was thought to be a normal part of aging and not everyone develops dementia as they grow older.

What causes Dementia?

It is the result of changes in certain regions of the brain that cause the neurons (nerve cells) and their connections to stop working properly. Researchers have connected changes in the brain to certain forms of dementia, but in most cases are unknown. For a small number of people, rare genetic variants that cause dementia have been identified.

Types of Dementia:

Dementia symptoms are progressive.

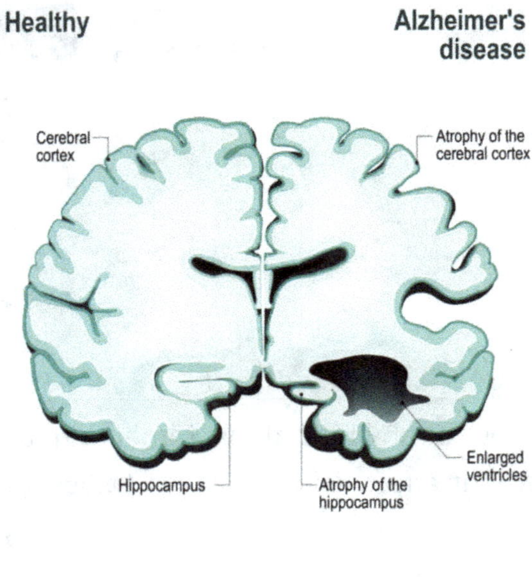

Figure 3 Alzheimer's Disease

1) Alzheimer's Disease:

It is caused by the buildup of amyloid plaques and tau tangles that kill nerve cells. It's not a normal part of aging, and while there's no cure, treatments and lifestyle changes can help manage symptoms.

Key Characteristics:

- Progressive: Symptoms worsen over time, starting with mild memory loss and progressing to severe cognitive decline.

- Irreversible: The damage to brain cells cannot be undone.

- Dementia: It's the leading cause of dementia, affecting 60-80% of cases.

Causes & What Happens in the Brain:

- Abnormal clumps of protein (amyloid plaques and tau tangles) form in the brain, disrupting nerve cell communication and leading to cell death.

- This process usually starts years before symptoms appear, often in the memory center of the brain (hippocampus).

2) Frontotemporal Dementia (FTD):

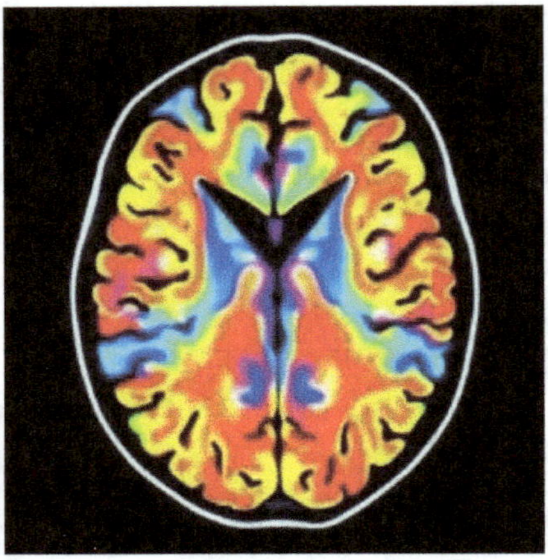

Figure 4 Frontotemporal Dementia (FTD)

Frontotemporal Dementia (FTD) is a group of progressive brain disorders causing nerve cell damage in the frontal and temporal lobes, leading to significant changes in personality, behavior, and language, often striking people between 45-64 years old. Symptoms vary but include apathy, impulsiveness, inappropriate social behavior, loss of empathy, or severe difficulty speaking, writing, and understanding language. It's an umbrella term for conditions like Behavior Variant FTD (bvFTD) and Primary Progressive Aphasia (PPA) that affect distinct functions but share the common root of frontal/temporal lobe atrophy.

Key Characteristics

• Location of Damage: primarily affects the brain's frontal lobes (behavior, judgment, movement) and temporal lobes (language, emotion).

• Typical Age: more common in younger adults (40s-60s) than other dementias like Alzheimer's.

• Progressive Nature: Symptoms worsen over time as more brain regions are affected.

Common Forms

• Behavioral Variant FTD (bvFTD): Changes personality, judgment, empathy, and conduct (e.g., impulsivity, apathy, inappropriate actions).

• Primary Progressive Aphasia (PPA): Impairs language, speech, reading, and writing.

• FTD-Related Movement Disorders: can cause stiffness, slow movement, or trouble with coordination

Symptoms

• Behavioral: socially inappropriate acts, apathy, loss of inhibition, compulsive behaviors, changes in appetite, poor hygiene, loss of empathy

Language: difficulty finding words, speaking fluently, understanding others, or writing

• Motor: stiff walking, clumsiness, muscle weakness, tremors (if movement disorders are present)

Causes & Diagnosis

• Caused by abnormal protein buildup (tau, TDP-43) in nerve cells, though genetics can play a role

• Diagnosis can be tricky as symptoms mimic psychiatric disorders, but early signs warrant a doctor visit.

3) Lewy body Dementia

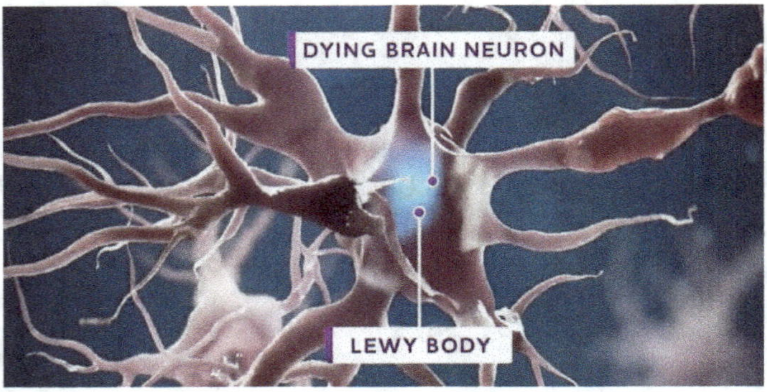

Figure 5 Lewy body Dementia Mustration showing neurons containing Lewy bodies small red spheres which are deposits of proteins accumulated in brain cells that cause their progressive degeneration

Dementia with Lewy bodies (DLB) is a progressive type of dementia that involves the formation of Lewy bodies in the nerve cells. DLB is the third most common cause of dementia, after Alzheimer's disease and vascular dementia. About 10 to 25 percent of all cases of dementia are due to DLB.

Lewy Body Dementia (LBD) and Parkinson's Disease Dementia (PDD) are related conditions characterized by abnormal protein clumps (Lewy bodies) in the brain, affecting thinking, movement, and behavior; the main difference is timing, with LBD showing dementia symptoms early alongside movement issues, while PDD develops dementia years after Parkinson's movement symptoms begin, both involving disrupted brain cell function from alpha-synuclein protein buildup.

Lewy Bodies

• What they are: tiny, abnormal clumps of the protein alpha-synuclein that build up in nerve cells, disrupting their function and eventually causing cell death

• Where they occur: in the brain's cortex and other areas, leading to symptoms of LBD and PDD

Dementia with Lewy Bodies (DLB)

Definition: A type of LBD where dementia (thinking problems like attention, memory, visual-spatial skills) appears early, often within a year of movement

Symptoms

- Visual hallucinations
- Movement symptoms
- Poor regulation of body functions
- Cognitive changes
- Trouble with sleep
- Varying attention
- Depression or apathy

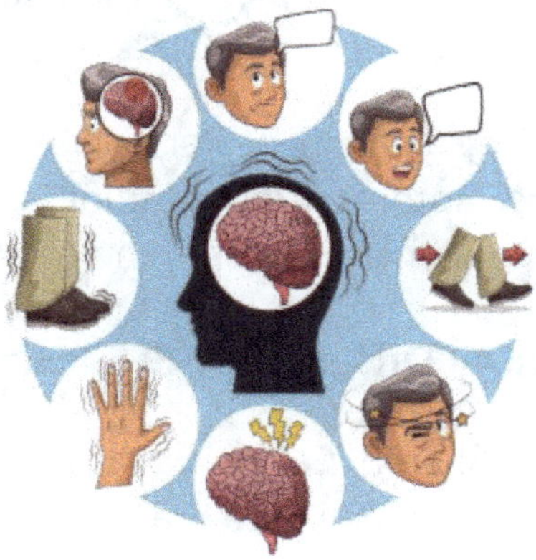

Key Features: Early visual hallucinations, fluctuating alertness, REM sleep disorder (acting out dreams), and Parkinson-like movement issues (rigidity, slow movement)

4) Parkinson's Disease Dementia (PDD)

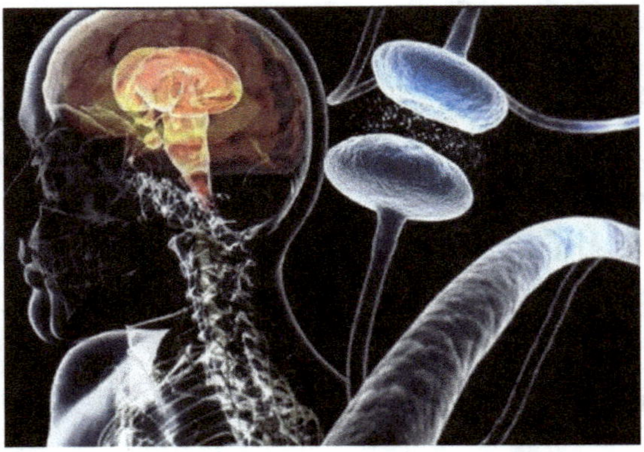

Figure 6 Parkinson's Disease Dementia (PDD)

Definition: Dementia that develops in someone who has had Parkinson's disease (a movement disorder) for at least a year

Key Features: Starts with classic Parkinson's movement symptoms (tremor, stiffness, shuffling walk) and progresses to dementia later in the disease course

Key Differences & Similarities (LBD vs. PDD)

• Shared Cause: Both involve Lewy bodies and loss of dopamine in the brain.

• Symptom onset: In DLB, cognitive and motor symptoms occur close together; in PDD, dementia develops much later after the movement disorder starts.

• Symptoms: Both have thinking issues, hallucinations, and motor problems, but hallucinations and cognitive fluctuations are more prominent and earlier in DLB.

5) Vascular Dementia

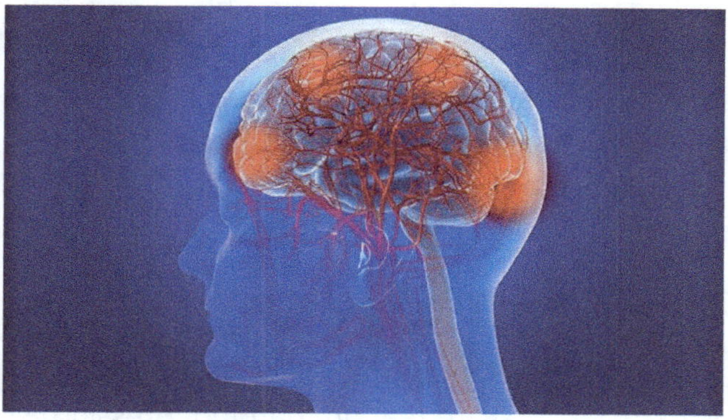

Figure 7 Vascular Dementia

Vascular dementia progresses through stages, often described as early (mild), middle (moderate), and late (severe), marked by increasing confusion, memory issues, and difficulty with daily tasks, though progression varies and can jump after strokes, with symptoms like trouble concentrating, language problems, and mood changes worsening over time, requiring more support until severe decline necessitates full-time care.

Stages

- **Early Stage (Mild):**

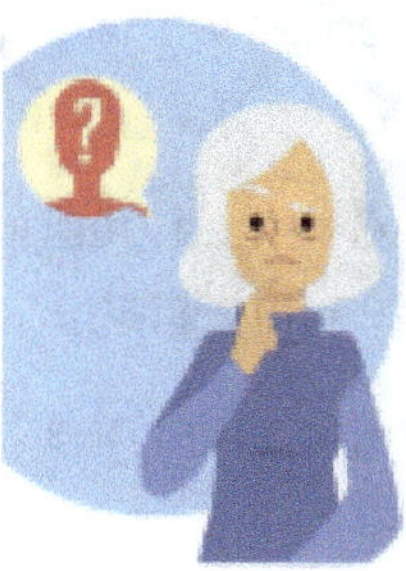

Subtle changes, mild confusion, difficulty with complex tasks, trouble with planning or organizing, but still independent

• **Middle Stage (Moderate):**

More significant decline, noticeable memory loss, communication difficulties, personality changes, trouble with daily tasks (cooking, bills), increased confusion, maybe sundowning

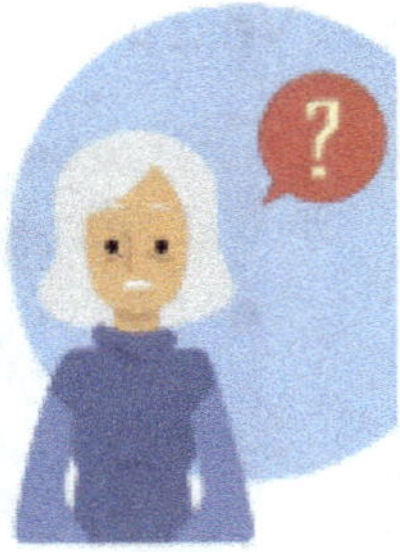

• **Late Stage (Severe):**

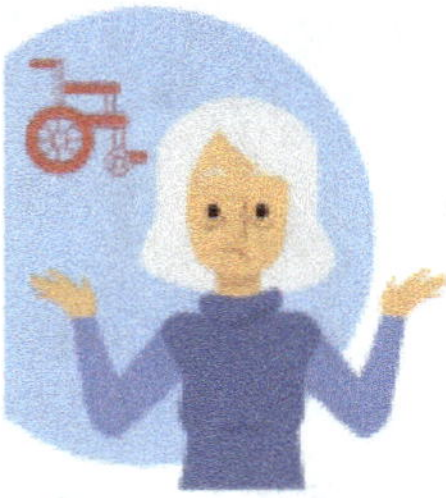

Major assistance needed for all self-care (eating, bathing, dressing), loss of most thinking skills, incontinence, severe confusion, requires 24/7 care

More Detailed (7-Stage Model)

1. Normal Behavior: No symptoms

2. Very Mild Changes: Slight confusion, mild attention/thinking issues

3. Mild Cognitive Decline: Symptoms noticeable to family (e.g., difficulty with complex tasks)

4. Moderate Cognitive Decline: Significant issues with daily tasks (cooking. managing finances)

5. Moderately Severe Decline: Difficulty remembering address/phone, dressing appropriately, often late-stage

6. Severe Decline: Incontinence, swallowing issues, needs daily help

7. Very Severe Decline: Requires constant, around-the-clock care

Key Characteristics

Variable Progression:

It can worsen suddenly after a stroke, or slowly; sometimes symptoms improve temporarily.

Stair-Step Pattern:

Often characterized by abrupt drops in function (like a stroke) followed by plateaus.

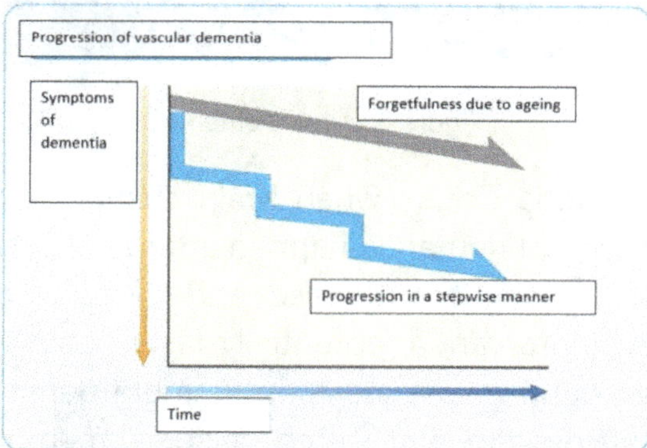

Symptoms

Memory loss, confusion, difficulty concentrating, impaired judgment, communication problems, mood changes, balance/mobility issues.

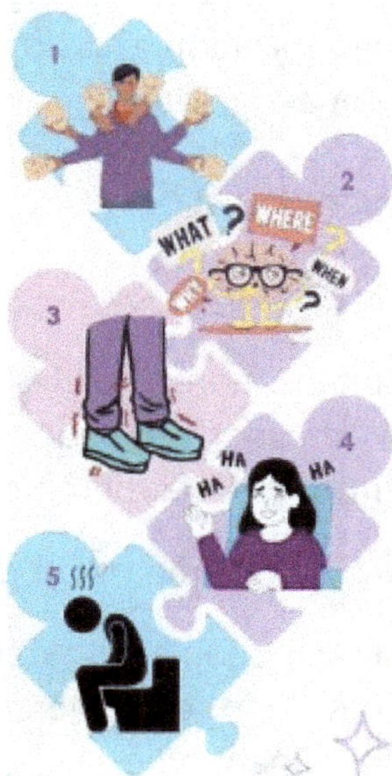

6) Mixed Dementia

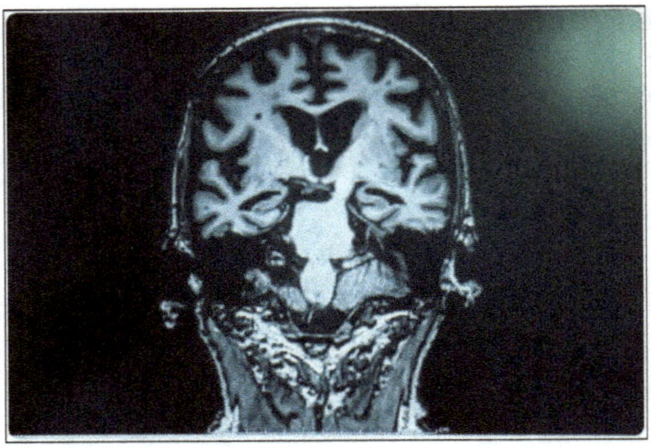

Figure 8 Mixed Dementia

Mixed dementia occurs when brain changes from more than one type of dementia happen at the same time, most commonly Alzheimer's disease and vascular dementia, leading to more varied, potentially faster, and harder-to-diagnose cognitive decline than a single dementia type. Symptoms overlap but often include memory issues (Alzheimer's) alongside problems with planning, organization, and slower thinking (vascular), making overall impact greater.

What is it?

Multiple pathologies:

Brain abnormalities from different dementias (like Alzheimer's plaques/tangles and blood vessel damage from vascular dementia, or Lewy bodies) coexist.

More common than diagnosed:

Many people with dementia, especially older adults, likely have mixed dementia, but it's often diagnosed as the dominant type.

Common combinations

- Alzheimer's disease + Vascular dementia (most common)
- Alzheimer's disease + Lewy body dementia
- Alzheimer's+ Vascular + Lewy Body dementia

Symptoms

Memory loss, confusion, disorientation: (from Alzheimer's)

• Difficulty with planning, organizing, decision-making, slower thinking, attention issues: (from vascular)

• Unsteady gait, restlessness, apathy, depression, and sometimes changes in urination

• Symptoms can be unpredictable, fluctuating, and worsen more rapidly.

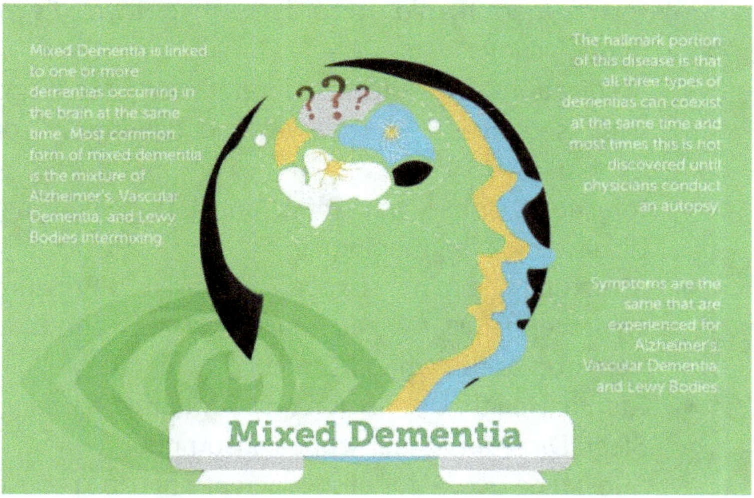

CHAPTER 2

REVERSIBLE CAUSES OF DEMENTIA

Reversible causes of dementia-like symptoms often stem from treatable conditions like depression, medication side effects, nutritional deficiencies (especially B12), thyroid problems, infections (UTIs, Lyme, Syphilis), sleep apnea, and alcohol/drug abuse, alongside structural issues like normal pressure hydrocephalus (NPH) or subdural hematomas (bleeding under the skull); early diagnosis is key to addressing these underlying issues and potentially reversing cognitive decline, notes UCI MIND.

Common Reversible Causes:

- Metabolic & Nutritional: Vitamin B12/B1/Folate deficiency, dehydration, electrolyte imbalance, thyroid/parathyroid disorders (hypothyroidism), hypoglycemia
- Medications: Side effects or interactions from drugs like sedatives, steroids, anticholinergics, or excessive alcohol
- Infections: Urinary tract infections (UTIs), HIV, Lyme disease, syphilis, meningitis
- Structural Brain Issues: Normal Pressure Hydrocephalus (NPH), brain tumors, subdural hematomas (bleeding from falls)
- Mental Health: Depression (pseudodementia)
- Sleep Disorders: Sleep apnea, insomnia
- Substance Use: Alcoholism, recreational drug abuse
- Heart/Lung Issues: Poor heart/lung function leading to lack of oxygen to the brain (hypoxia)

When to Suspect a Reversible Cause:

Look for rapid decline, fluctuating symptoms, younger age of onset, or a history of high-risk behaviors or recent injuries (like falls). An accurate evaluation by a doctor is crucial for identifying and treating these potentially reversible conditions, preventing misdiagnosis as progressive dementia like Alzheimer's Disease.

There are over 100 conditions that cause dementia, but four main types account for most cases: Alzheimer's Disease, the most common; Vascular Dementia, from blood flow issues; Lewy Body Dementia, involving protein deposits (Lewy bodies); and Frontotemporal Dementia, affecting personality and behavior.

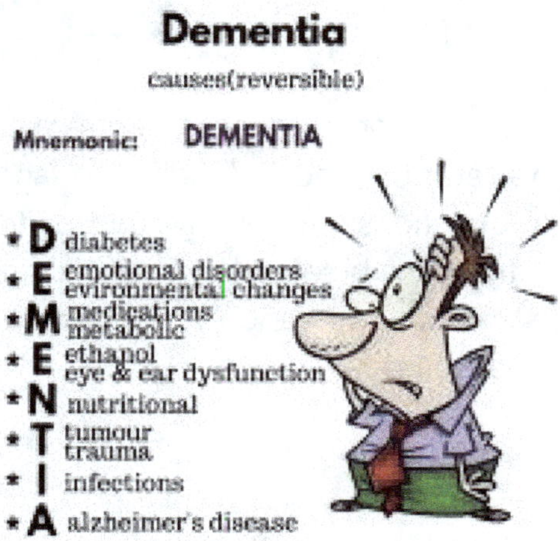

CHAPTER 3

HOW TO COMMUNICATE WITH PEOPLE WITH DEMENTIA?

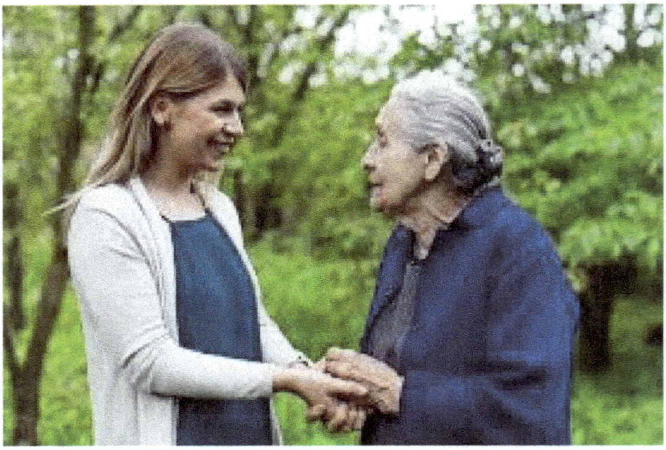

Use simple words, short sentences, and a calm tone; get to their eye level and use touch /body language to connect; use "yes/no" questions and reminisce to build connection. Minimize distractions break tasks into steps; and focus on reassurance, validation, and redirection rather than correcting or arguing.

The "4R's" Approach:

Use the 4 Rs of Dementia Care:

Reassure: Calm their fears.

Reconsider: See things from their perspective.

Redirect: Shift their focus.

Relax: Stay Calm yourself.

*Enter Their Reality: Instead of correcting or arguing when they are confused, validate their feelings. If they think it is 1970, ask then about their day in that year rather than trying to "bring them back" to the present.

*Non-Verbal Mastery: Because verbal processing declines, your body language, eye contact, and tone of voice become more important than your words. Use gentle touch and a calm, low pitched voice to convey safety.

Simplify Requests: Ask "yes" or "no" questions instead of open-ended ones ("Would you like tea?"* instead of *"What do you want to drink?"*)

Behavioral Management Skills:

Behaviors like wandering, agitation, or "sundowning" (late-day confusion) are often forms of communication for unmet needs.

*Identify Triggers: Learn to "investigate the cause of a behavior. Agitation might be triggered by loud noises, pain, or hunger.

*Environmental Modifications: Skillfully adjust the home by reducing clutter, improving lighting to reduce shadows (which can look like hallucinations), and using safety locks to prevent wandering.

*Routine Building: Creating a predictable daily schedule for meals, showers, and sleep helps reduce anxiety and provides a sense of security.

Emotional Resilience & Self-Care:

The most critical skill is often "caregiver Mastery" —the ability to care for oneself to avoid burnout.

*Boundary Setting: learning to say "no" to extra responsibilities and delegating tasks like grocery shopping or medication pick-up to others

*Emotional Reframing: separating the disease from the person; recognizing that aggression is a symptom of the disease, not a personal attack, helps maintain compassion

*Utilizing Resources: proactively seeking Respite Care through adult day programs or in-home aids to ensure you have time to rest

Verbal Communication Strategies:

Keep it Simple: Use short, clear sentences and familiar words. Avoid abstract concepts or complex instructions.

Be Clear & Direct: State one idea at a time. Instead of *"Let's get ready, go to the doctor, then the store,"* say, *"We're going to the doctor now".*

Speak Slowly & Calmly: Use a lower pitch and a reassuring tone, not louder volume, which can sound like yelling.

Ask Simple Questions: Use yes/no questions (*"Would you like coffee?"*) instead of open-ended ones.

Repeat & Rephrase: If they don't understand, repeat the exact same words first; if still unclear, rephrase patiently.

Nonverbal & Environmental Cues:

Get on their level: Move to eye level to help them focus and reduce intimidation.

Use Touch: A gentle touch (hand holding) can be very reassuring and connect when words fail.

Minimize Distractions: Turn off the TV/radio and move to a quiet space.

Be aware of Body Language: Your expressions and posture matter; be patient and positive.

Interaction Techniques:

Don't Argue or Correct: Validate their feelings; redirect their attention if they become upset

Listen Actively: Pay attention to their tone and gestures; they're still communicating emotions

Break Down Tasks: For activities, offer clear, one-step instructions (*"Put your arm here").*

Reminisce: Talk about the past, as long term memories are often intact and soothing.

Key Mindset:

Patient & Empathy: Remember they are struggling; focus on connection, not perfection.

Reassure & Redirect: Reassure then they are safe and redirect to a positive focus when needed.

Here are 20 things to say, focusing on positive communication:

- *"I understand that's how you remember it."* (instead of *"That's wrong."*)
- *"It's so nice to spend time with you."*
- *"Let's talk about what you are feeling right now."*
- *"I'm sorry, I forgot."* (when accepting blame on a perceived mistake)
- *"Tell me more about that."* (instead of asking *"Do you remember?"*)

Connection & Presence:

1. "I remember our beach trips. The water was so blue." (sharing a memory)
2. "What a lovely day it is." (focusing on the present)
3. "This is (your name). I'm here to help." (simple instructions)
4. "I love it when we......" (sharing positive, familiar activities)
5. "Would you like some milk and cookies? Chocolate chip or oatmeal?" (simple choices)

Redirection & Comfort:

a) *"Let's go for a walk."* (gentle redirection)
b) *"How about we look at these pictures?"* (using prompt like photos)
c) *"You look wonderful!"* (positive, simple compliment)
d) *"It's okay, let's figure it out together."* (collaborative support)
e) *"He'll be here for dinner."* (If they're asking for someone, reassure them.)

Simple & Direct:

a) *"Please put your shoes on."* (clear, simple instruction)

b) *"Here is your hat."* (direct description)

c) *"Let's go here."* (reassurance if they're anxious)

d) *"I'm here with you."* (simple, reassuring presence)

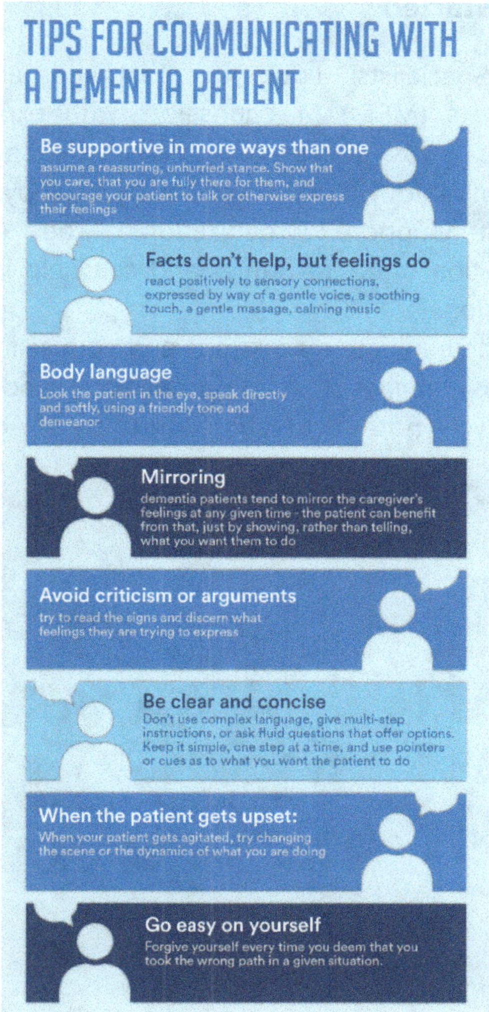

CHAPTER 4

HOW TO BUILD A RELATIONSHIP WITH SOMEONE WHO HAS DEMENTIA?

Getting Started

- Seek Specialists: Look for Marriage and Family Therapists (MFTs) or counselors with experience in chronic Illness, dementia, or elder care, suggests the Association for Marriage and Family Therapy.
- Contact Support Organizations: The Alzheimer's Association offers resources and can help locate local professionals.
- Start Early: Initiate discussions and counseling early, as it helps families manage transitions and decisions proactively, notes the National Institute of Aging (NIA).

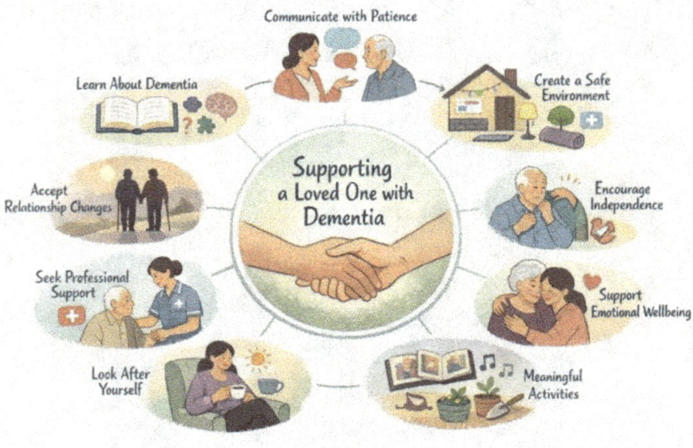
Communicate with Patience
Learn About Dementia
Create a Safe Environment
Supporting a Loved One with Dementia
Accept Relationship Changes
Encourage Independence
Seek Professional Support
Support Emotional Wellbeing
Look After Yourself
Meaningful Activities

Dealing with a loved one diagnosed with dementia can present some unique challenges to family caregivers. Dementia can affect everyday tasks, communication skills, and even temper and personality, causing major disruption to the daily lives of both caregiver and loved one.

As your loved one's condition progresses, the amount of time you may need to spend assisting them will increase as well. Not only can this affect other major aspects of your life such as your job or kids, but it can also be financially draining.

Being able to connect on a meaningful level while caring for someone with dementia is incredibly vital. A strong relationship can create tight bonds and even reduce the symptoms of dementia in your loved one. Understanding dementia and learning how to create a meaningful relationship with your loved one is something you have to continue to develop with patience and effort over time.

5 Ways to Keep Growing Your Relationship with Your Loved One with Dementia:

1. **Find an activity or hobby you both enjoy:**
   A great way to bond is to find a hobby or activity that both you and your loved one can participate in together. It can be an activity as simple as sitting and knitting or as engaging as joining a club. Whatever it might be, make sure it's something you both look forward to and enjoy.

2. **Be patient and adapt to their level of communication:**
   Communication can become limited as the disease progresses, and your loved one might have a hard time trying to form ideas or carry on a conversation. Due to this, they might experience social withdrawal as well.

It's important for you to be patient and adapt to their level of communication.

3. **Take care of yourself:**
   Although this might not be an obvious tip, actually taking care of yourself, both physically and mentally, can have a drastic impact on your relationship with your loved one. By practicing self-care, you will be able to be your best self, and thus, create a strong and meaningful bond with your loved one.

4. **Non-verbal communication:**
   As communication between you and your loved one changes, you might consider relying on more non-verbal communication cues to interact with them. Understanding dementia and the ways it will affect your ability to interact with them is a huge step in creating a strong, meaningful relationship. A warm hug or pat on the shoulder can be positive examples of non-verbal communication that will mean a lot to your loved one.

5. **Cherish old memories while creating new ones:**
   Being able to reminisce about past events your loved one might remember fondly is a great way to bond. Additionally, don't just remember "the old days," but also create new memories right now by spending quality time together regularly. Indulging with your loved one and appreciating the relationship you have now can help your bond grow stronger.

CHAPTER 5

IS FAMILY COUNSELING NECESSARY FOR A CAREGIVER?

Benefits of Family Counseling

Family Counseling helps navigate communication challenges, manage emotional stress, resolve conflicts over care, and adjust to role changes, improving overall family well-being and caregiving effectiveness. Association for Marriage and Family Therapy (AAMFT) and the Alzheimer's Association. Improved Communication: Learn new verbal and non-verbal techniques to connect with the person with dementia and with each other. Association for Marriage and Family Therapy (AAMFT) and the Alzheimer's Association.

• Emotional Support: Process of feeling of anger, guilt, sadness, and grief that arise from the complex loss associated with dementia, says Association for Marriage and Family Therapy (AAMFT) and the Alzheimer's Association.

Conflict Resolution: Smooth out disagreements about caregiving responsibilities, finances, and decision making, according to the AAMFT.

• Education & Preparation: Understand the disease's progression and learn effective management strategies from experts, mentions the NIH.

• Reduced Caregiver Burden: Develop coping mechanisms for stress and frustration, protecting the mental and physical health of caregiver, notes MedlinePlus and the fisher Center for Alzheimer's research Foundation.

When to Seek Counseling:

• Signs of Depression/Anxiety: persistent sadness, loss of interest, excessive worry, or changes in sleep/appetite

• Overwhelm & Burnout: feeling constantly exhausted, resentful, or like you're losing control

Difficulty Coping: struggling to manage daily tasks or feeling isolated

• Grief & Loss: experiencing anticipatory grief or profound loss after the loved one's death

Alternatives & Supplements:

• Support Groups: offer peer connection but lack individual depth

• Respite Care: provides breaks but doesn't address emotional trauma

• Psychiatrist: may be needed for medication in severe cases

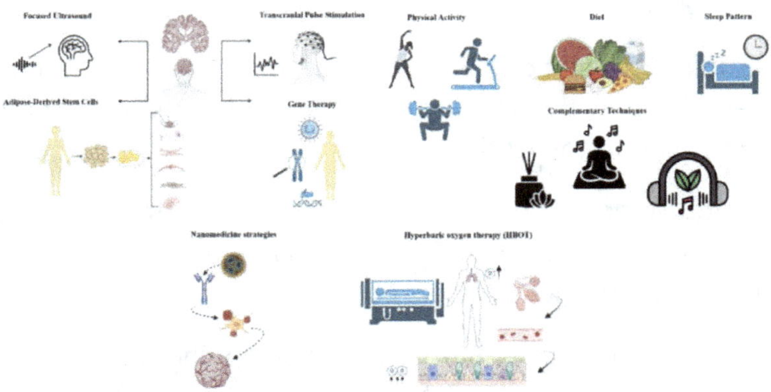

CHAPTER 6

IS COUNSELING NECESSARY FOR A CAREGIVER?

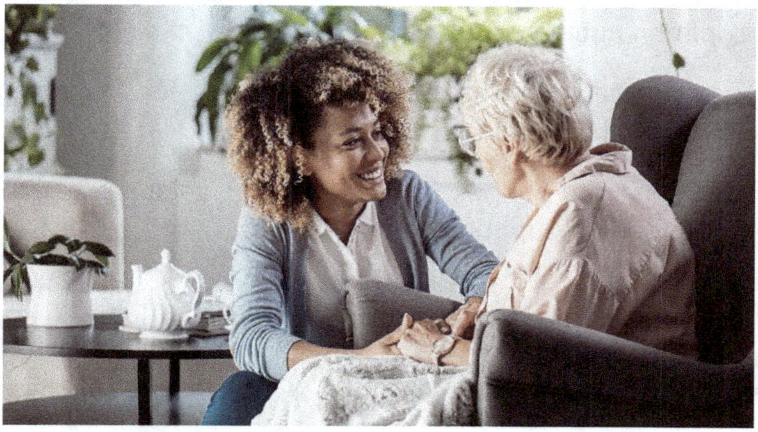

Benefits of 1 to 1 Counseling

One to One counseling is often crucial for caregivers. It provides Vital emotional support, coping strategies, tools to manage guilt, anxiety, burnout, and grief, helping them maintain their wellbeing while navigating the immense challenges of caregiving, and preventing serious mental health issues like depression. It's highly recommended to process complex emotions, develop new perspectives, and learn healthier ways to respond to stress, ultimately improving both the caregiver's and care recipient's quality of life.

• Emotional Processing: a safe space to work through feelings like anger, guilt, fear, helplessness, and anticipatory grief

• Skill Building: Learn coping mechanisms, stress management techniques, and how to set boundaries.

• Reframing Thoughts: Challenge negative thought patterns (cognitive Behavioral Therapy—CBT) and find new ways to manage the situation.

• Preventing Burnout & Depression: proactively addresses caregiver burnout and can prevent clinical depression, a common outcome.

• Crisis Management: Develop strategies for managing difficult behaviors and emotional stress.

• Personalized Support: tailored to your unique situation, unlike general support groups

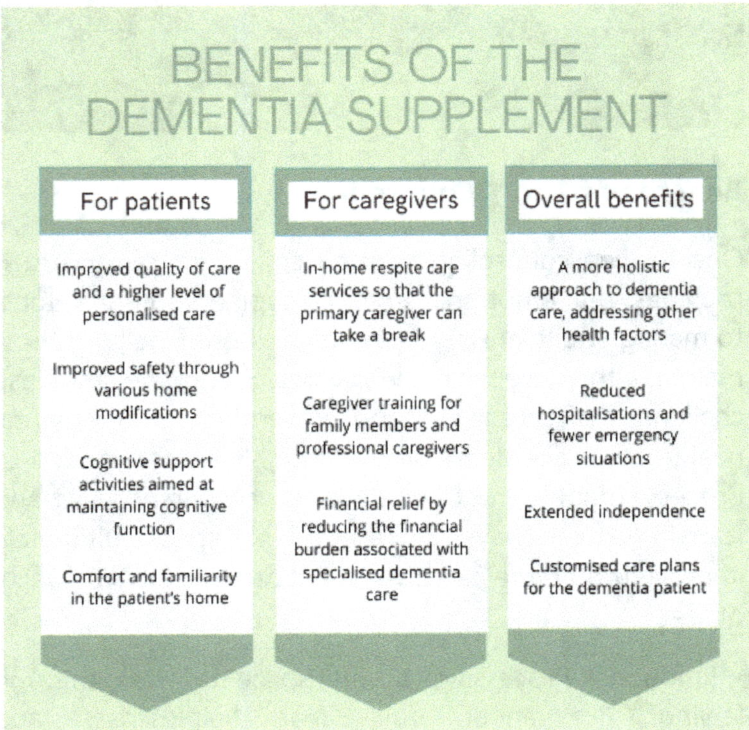

ALL ABOUT MARIA

Maria Cianciolo, CADDCT, CDP, APDA

Maria is a lifelong Connecticut resident and currently lives in the small town of Prospect. She loves her family and enjoys fitness, fishing, baking, reading, writing and "classic movies" just to name a few.

Maria has been in the Health Care Field since 1993 with a particular passion for Seniors. She has always been and continues to be personally involved in their wellbeing. Her commitment to providing the BEST "quality of life" is second to none. She is deeply committed to advocating for seniors in her community.

She is nationally certified as a "Dementia Care Practitioner & Educator" which enables her to professionally tailor resident programs and educate associates. She is also a "Parkinson's Awareness Trainer" with great successes in personalized resident programs. These include assessment and implementation of sparring, balance strategies, and cognitive skills.

Maria is very involved in community outreach with a special attention to Veteran's Affairs, the American Cancer Society, the Heart Association and the Alzheimer's Association. Her creativity, enthusiasm, and energy are some of her strongest attributes.

Her personal work with Family Members & Caregivers through both individual and group counseling is always a priority, which in turn builds a strong sense of unity and support within the Memory Care community.

She's also the recipient of CALA's "Humanitarian of the Year Award for her relief work in Florida during "Hurricane Ian".

She's been a featured guest along with Teepa Snow & Dr. Macie Smith on "Dementia Diva's", both the Pilot Episode & Episode 2. Produced by Caregiving & Arts.

NOTE FROM MARIA

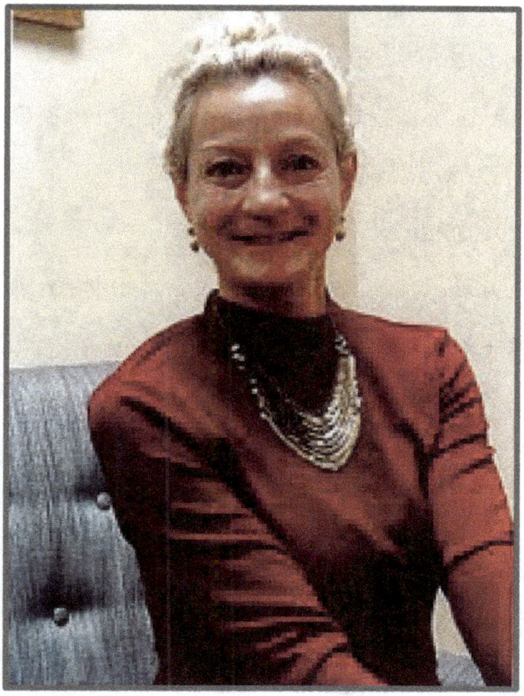

Over the course of my career, it's been apparent that a practical, daily use handbook is needed "in the field" for quick reference. I particularly noted this from my experience working alongside Certified Nursing Assistants & family caregivers, witnessing the daily struggles and hardships that come with being a "Dementia Caregiver," especially those with very little understanding of the disease. There is a tremendous need for a handbook with "Quick Reference" answers—on the spot. Therefore, I wrote this handbook for Dementia Caregivers that will educate, offer quick solutions, manage strategies, and communication techniques to help them connect & establish life-long bonds with individuals with Dementia.

REFERENCES

- **Introduction:**

Why write a resource guide for Family Members & Caregivers?

Reference: Oxford Language

Why title the guide "Kaleidoscope"?

Reference: Alzheimer's Association, Merriam Webster Dictionary

- **Chapter 1: What is Dementia?**

Reference: Alzheimer's Association, Alz.org

What Causes Dementia?

Reference: Mayo Clinic

3. Types of Dementia

A) Alzheimer's Disease

B) Frontotemporal Dementia

C) Lewy body Dementia

D) Parkinson's Dementia

E) Key Differences & Similarities (LBD vs. PDD)

F) Vascular Dementia

G) Mixed Dementia, what is It?

Reference: The National Institute of Aging (NIH), Alzheimer's Assoc.org, Alz.org

- **Chapter 2: Reversible Causes of Dementia:**

Reference: Mind.UCi.edu, NIH, PubMed Central

- **Chapter 3: How to Communicate with people who have Dementia?**

Reference: Alz.org, Alzheimer's Assoc.org

A) The "4 R's" Approach

B) Behavioral Management Skills

C) Verbal Communication Strategies

D) Interaction Techniques

E) Key Mindset

F) 20 Things to say, focusing on positive Communication

G) Connection & Presence

H) Redirection & Comfort

I) Simple & Direct

- **Chapter 4: How to build a relationship with someone who has Dementia?**

Reference: Alz.org, saintsimeons.org

- **Chapter 5: Is Family Counseling necessary for a caregiver?**

Reference: Association for Marriage and Family Therapy (AAMFT), Alz.org, NIH, Medline & Fisher Center for Alzheimer's Research Foundation

- **Chapter 6: Is Counseling necessary for a caregiver?**

Reference: AgingCare.com, Conseling.org, National Institute of Health (NIH)